M000091903

THIS JOURNAL BELONGS TO:

_____

Copyright © 2019 Enchanted Willow. All rights reserved. No part of this publication may be resold, hired out, transmitted or reproduced in any form by any electronic or mechanical means including photocopying, recording, or information storage and retrieval without prior written authority from the publishers.

PROGRESS
TRACKER

What to Track	Week 1	Week 2
Weight		
Chest		
Hips		
Arms		
Thighs		

What to Track	Week 3	Week 4	Week 5	Week 6
Weight				
Chest				
Hips				
Arms				
Thighs				
What to Track	Week 7	Week 8	Week 8	Week 10
Weight				
Chest				
Hips				
Arms				
Thighs				
What to Track	Week 11	Week 12	Week 13	Week 14
Weight				
Chest				
Hips				
Arms				
Thighs				

Date: _____ Fasting Day?　Y　N

		MACROS	
BREAKFAST		Protein	
		Carbs	
		Fat	
		Calories	
LUNCH		MACROS	
		Protein	
		Carbs	
		Fat	
		Calories	
DINNER		MACROS	
		Protein	
		Carbs	
		Fat	
		Calories	
SNACKS		MACROS	
		Protein	
		Carbs	
		Fat	
		Calories	

Hunger / Cravings

Hydration

Today's Weight

Notes / Observations

....
....
....
....
....
....
....
....
....

Today I Feel...

Sleep Quality

Sleep Time

_____

Wake Time

_____

Date: _____   Fasting Day?   Y   N

		MACROS	
BREAKFAST		Protein	
		Carbs	
		Fat	
		Calories	
LUNCH		MACROS	
		Protein	
		Carbs	
		Fat	
		Calories	
DINNER		MACROS	
		Protein	
		Carbs	
		Fat	
		Calories	
SNACKS		MACROS	
		Protein	
		Carbs	
		Fat	
		Calories	

Hunger / Cravings

Some
None   Intense

Hydration

Today's Weight

Notes / Observations

....
....
....
....
....
....
....
....
....

Today I Feel...

Sleep Quality

Sleep Time

_____

Wake Time

_____

Date: _____ Fasting Day?   Y   N

		MACROS	
BREAKFAST		Protein	
		Carbs	
		Fat	
		Calories	
LUNCH		MACROS	
		Protein	
		Carbs	
		Fat	
		Calories	
DINNER		MACROS	
		Protein	
		Carbs	
		Fat	
		Calories	
SNACKS		MACROS	
		Protein	
		Carbs	
		Fat	
		Calories	

Hunger / Cravings

Some

None   Intense

Hydration

Today's Weight

Notes / Observations

....

....

....

....

....

....

....

....

....

Today I Feel...

Sleep Quality

Sleep Time

_____

Wake Time

_____

zZz

Date: _____ Fasting Day?   Y   N

	MACROS	
BREAKFAST	Protein	
	Carbs	
	Fat	
	Calories	
	MACROS	
LUNCH	Protein	
	Carbs	
	Fat	
	Calories	
	MACROS	
DINNER	Protein	
	Carbs	
	Fat	
	Calories	
	MACROS	
SNACKS	Protein	
	Carbs	
	Fat	
	Calories	

Hunger / Cravings

Some

None   Intense

Hydration

Today's Weight

Notes / Observations

....

....

....

....

....

....

....

....

Today I Feel...

Sleep Quality

Sleep Time

_____

Wake Time

_____

Date: _____   Fasting Day?   Y   N

		MACROS	
BREAKFAST		Protein	
		Carbs	
		Fat	
		Calories	
LUNCH		MACROS	
		Protein	
		Carbs	
		Fat	
		Calories	
DINNER		MACROS	
		Protein	
		Carbs	
		Fat	
		Calories	
SNACKS		MACROS	
		Protein	
		Carbs	
		Fat	
		Calories	

Hunger / Cravings

Some

None   Intense

Hydration

Today's Weight

Notes / Observations

Today I Feel...

Sleep Quality

Sleep Time
_____

Wake Time
_____

Date: _____   Fasting Day?   Y   N

		MACROS	
BREAKFAST		Protein	
		Carbs	
		Fat	
		Calories	
LUNCH		MACROS	
		Protein	
		Carbs	
		Fat	
		Calories	
DINNER		MACROS	
		Protein	
		Carbs	
		Fat	
		Calories	
SNACKS		MACROS	
		Protein	
		Carbs	
		Fat	
		Calories	

Hunger / Cravings

Some

None   Intense

Hydration

Today's Weight

Notes / Observations

....
....
....
....
....
....
....
....
....

Today I Feel...

Sleep Quality

Sleep Time

_____

Wake Time

_____

Date: _____   Fasting Day?   Y   N

BREAKFAST		MACROS	
		Protein	.
		Carbs	
		Fat	
		Calories	

Hunger / Cravings

LUNCH		MACROS	
		Protein	
		Carbs	
		Fat	
		Calories	

Hydration

DINNER		MACROS	
		Protein	
		Carbs	
		Fat	
		Calories	

Today's Weight

SNACKS		MACROS	
		Protein	
		Carbs	
		Fat	
		Calories	

Notes / Observations

....
....
....
....
....
....
....
....
....

Today I Feel...

Sleep Quality

Sleep Time

_____

Wake Time

_____

Date: _____ Fasting Day? Y N

		MACROS	
BREAKFAST		Protein	
		Carbs	
		Fat	
		Calories	
LUNCH		MACROS	
		Protein	
		Carbs	
		Fat	
		Calories	
DINNER		MACROS	
		Protein	
		Carbs	
		Fat	
		Calories	
SNACKS		MACROS	
		Protein	
		Carbs	
		Fat	
		Calories	

Hunger / Cravings

Some

None   Intense

Hydration

Today's Weight

Notes / Observations

....
....
....
....
....
....
....
....
....
....

Today I Feel...

Sleep Quality

Sleep Time

_____

Wake Time

_____

Date: _____ Fasting Day?   Y   N

BREAKFAST		Macros	
		Protein	
		Carbs	
		Fat	
		Calories	
LUNCH		Macros	
		Protein	
		Carbs	
		Fat	
		Calories	
DINNER		Macros	
		Protein	
		Carbs	
		Fat	
		Calories	
SNACKS		Macros	
		Protein	
		Carbs	
		Fat	
		Calories	

Hunger / Cravings

Hydration

Today's Weight

Notes / Observations

....
....
....
....
....
....
....
....
....

Today I Feel...

Sleep Quality

Sleep Time

_____

Wake Time

_____

Date: _____   Fasting Day?   Y   N

		MACROS	
BREAKFAST		Protein	
		Carbs	
		Fat	
		Calories	
LUNCH		MACROS	
		Protein	
		Carbs	
		Fat	
		Calories	
DINNER		MACROS	
		Protein	
		Carbs	
		Fat	
		Calories	
SNACKS		MACROS	
		Protein	
		Carbs	
		Fat	
		Calories	

Hunger / Cravings

Some
None   Intense

Hydration

Today's Weight

Notes / Observations

....

....

....

....

....

....

....

....

....

....

Today I Feel...

Sleep Quality

Sleep Time

_____

Wake Time

_____

Date: _____ Fasting Day?   Y   N

		MACROS	
BREAKFAST		Protein	
		Carbs	
		Fat	
		Calories	
LUNCH		MACROS	
		Protein	
		Carbs	
		Fat	
		Calories	
DINNER		MACROS	
		Protein	
		Carbs	
		Fat	
		Calories	
SNACKS		MACROS	
		Protein	
		Carbs	
		Fat	
		Calories	

Hunger / Cravings

Some

None   Intense

Hydration

Today's Weight

Notes / Observations

....
....
....
....
....
....
....
....
....

Today I Feel...

Sleep Quality

Sleep Time
_____

Wake Time
_____

Date: _____   Fasting Day?   Y   N

	MACROS	
BREAKFAST	Protein	
	Carbs	
	Fat	
	Calories	
	MACROS	
LUNCH	Protein	
	Carbs	
	Fat	
	Calories	
	MACROS	
DINNER	Protein	
	Carbs	
	Fat	
	Calories	
	MACROS	
SNACKS	Protein	
	Carbs	
	Fat	
	Calories	

Hunger / Cravings

Some

None   Intense

Hydration

Today's Weight

Notes / Observations

....

....

....

....

....

....

....

....

....

Today I Feel...

Sleep Quality

Sleep Time

_____

Wake Time

_____

Date: _____ Fasting Day?   Y   N

	MACROS	
BREAKFAST	Protein	
	Carbs	
	Fat	
	Calories	
	MACROS	
LUNCH	Protein	
	Carbs	
	Fat	
	Calories	
	MACROS	
DINNER	Protein	
	Carbs	
	Fat	
	Calories	
	MACROS	
SNACKS	Protein	
	Carbs	
	Fat	
	Calories	

Hunger / Cravings

Some
None   Intense

Hydration

Today's Weight

Notes / Observations

....
....
....
....
....
....
....
....
....

Today I Feel...

Sleep Quality

Sleep Time
_____

Wake Time
_____

Date: _____   Fasting Day?   Y   N

BREAKFAST		Macros	
		Protein	
		Carbs	
		Fat	
		Calories	

LUNCH		Macros	
		Protein	
		Carbs	
		Fat	
		Calories	

DINNER		Macros	
		Protein	
		Carbs	
		Fat	
		Calories	

SNACKS		Macros	
		Protein	
		Carbs	
		Fat	
		Calories	

Hunger / Cravings

None   Some   Intense

Hydration

Today's Weight

Notes / Observations

....
....
....
....
....
....
....
....
....

Today I Feel...

Sleep Quality

Sleep Time

_____

Wake Time

_____

Date: _____   Fasting Day?   Y   N

		MACROS	
BREAKFAST		Protein	
		Carbs	
		Fat	
		Calories	
LUNCH		MACROS	
		Protein	
		Carbs	
		Fat	
		Calories	
DINNER		MACROS	
		Protein	
		Carbs	
		Fat	
		Calories	
SNACKS		MACROS	
		Protein	
		Carbs	
		Fat	
		Calories	

Hunger / Cravings

Some

None   Intense

Hydration

Today's Weight

Notes / Observations

....
....
....
....
....
....
....
....
....

Today I Feel...

Sleep Quality

Sleep Time
_____

Wake Time
_____

Date: _____   Fasting Day?   Y   N

		MACROS	
BREAKFAST		Protein	
		Carbs	
		Fat	
		Calories	
LUNCH		MACROS	
		Protein	
		Carbs	
		Fat	
		Calories	
DINNER		MACROS	
		Protein	
		Carbs	
		Fat	
		Calories	
SNACKS		MACROS	
		Protein	
		Carbs	
		Fat	
		Calories	

Hunger / Cravings

Some

None   Intense

Hydration

Today's Weight

Notes / Observations

....

....

....

....

....

....

....

....

....

Today I Feel...

Sleep Quality

Sleep Time

_____

Wake Time

_____

Date: _____   Fasting Day?   Y   N

		MACROS	
BREAKFAST		Protein	
		Carbs	
		Fat	
		Calories	
LUNCH		MACROS	
		Protein	
		Carbs	
		Fat	
		Calories	
DINNER		MACROS	
		Protein	
		Carbs	
		Fat	
		Calories	
SNACKS		MACROS	
		Protein	
		Carbs	
		Fat	
		Calories	

Hunger / Cravings

Some

None   Intense

Hydration

Today's Weight

Notes / Observations

....
....
....
....
....
....
....
....
....

Today I Feel...

Sleep Quality

Sleep Time
_____

Wake Time
_____

Date: _____   Fasting Day?   Y   N

		MACROS	
BREAKFAST		Protein	
		Carbs	
		Fat	
		Calories	
LUNCH		MACROS	
		Protein	
		Carbs	
		Fat	
		Calories	
DINNER		MACROS	
		Protein	
		Carbs	
		Fat	
		Calories	
SNACKS		MACROS	
		Protein	
		Carbs	
		Fat	
		Calories	

Hunger / Cravings

Some
None   Intense

Hydration

Today's Weight

Notes / Observations

....
....
....
....
....
....
....
....
....
....

Today I Feel...

Sleep Quality

Sleep Time

_____

Wake Time

_____

Date: _____   Fasting Day?   Y   N

BREAKFAST		MACROS	
		Protein	
		Carbs	
		Fat	
		Calories	
LUNCH		MACROS	
		Protein	
		Carbs	
		Fat	
		Calories	
DINNER		MACROS	
		Protein	
		Carbs	
		Fat	
		Calories	
SNACKS		MACROS	
		Protein	
		Carbs	
		Fat	
		Calories	

Hunger / Cravings

Hydration

Today's Weight

Notes / Observations

....
....
....
....
....
....
....
....
....

Today I Feel...

Sleep Quality

Sleep Time
_____

Wake Time
_____

Date: _____   Fasting Day?   Y   N

		MACROS	
BREAKFAST		Protein	
		Carbs	
		Fat	
		Calories	
LUNCH		MACROS	
		Protein	
		Carbs	
		Fat	
		Calories	
DINNER		MACROS	
		Protein	
		Carbs	
		Fat	
		Calories	
SNACKS		MACROS	
		Protein	
		Carbs	
		Fat	
		Calories	

Hunger / Cravings

Hydration

Today's Weight

Notes / Observations

....
....
....
....
....
....
....
....
....

Today I Feel...

Sleep Quality

Sleep Time

_____

Wake Time

_____

Date: _____   Fasting Day?   Y   N

		MACROS	
BREAKFAST		Protein	
		Carbs	
		Fat	
		Calories	
LUNCH		MACROS	
		Protein	
		Carbs	
		Fat	
		Calories	
DINNER		MACROS	
		Protein	
		Carbs	
		Fat	
		Calories	
SNACKS		MACROS	
		Protein	
		Carbs	
		Fat	
		Calories	

Hunger / Cravings

Some

None   Intense

Hydration

Today's Weight

Notes / Observations

....

....

....

....

....

....

....

....

....

Today I Feel...

Sleep Quality

Sleep Time

_____

Wake Time

_____

Date: _____   Fasting Day?   Y   N

	MACROS	
BREAKFAST	Protein	
	Carbs	
	Fat	
	Calories	
	MACROS	
LUNCH	Protein	
	Carbs	
	Fat	
	Calories	
	MACROS	
DINNER	Protein	
	Carbs	
	Fat	
	Calories	
	MACROS	
SNACKS	Protein	
	Carbs	
	Fat	
	Calories	

Hunger / Cravings

Some

None   Intense

Hydration

Today's Weight

Notes / Observations

....

....

....

....

....

....

....

....

....

....

....

Today I Feel...

Sleep Quality

Sleep Time

_____

Wake Time

_____

Date: _____   Fasting Day?   Y   N

	MACROS	
BREAKFAST	Protein	
	Carbs	
	Fat	
	Calories	
	MACROS	
LUNCH	Protein	
	Carbs	
	Fat	
	Calories	
	MACROS	
DINNER	Protein	
	Carbs	
	Fat	
	Calories	
	MACROS	
SNACKS	Protein	
	Carbs	
	Fat	
	Calories	

Hunger / Cravings

Hydration

Today's Weight

Notes / Observations

Today I Feel...

Sleep Quality

Sleep Time

_____

Wake Time

_____

Date: _____   Fasting Day?   Y   N

		MACROS	
BREAKFAST		Protein	
		Carbs	
		Fat	
		Calories	
LUNCH		MACROS	
		Protein	
		Carbs	
		Fat	
		Calories	
DINNER		MACROS	
		Protein	
		Carbs	
		Fat	
		Calories	
SNACKS		MACROS	
		Protein	
		Carbs	
		Fat	
		Calories	

Hunger / Cravings

Some
None   Intense

Hydration

Today's Weight

Notes / Observations

....

....

....

....

....

....

....

....

....

....

Today I Feel...

Sleep Quality

Sleep Time
_____

Wake Time
_____

Date: _____ Fasting Day?   Y   N

		MACROS	
BREAKFAST		Protein	
		Carbs	
		Fat	
		Calories	
LUNCH		MACROS	
		Protein	
		Carbs	
		Fat	
		Calories	
DINNER		MACROS	
		Protein	
		Carbs	
		Fat	
		Calories	
SNACKS		MACROS	
		Protein	
		Carbs	
		Fat	
		Calories	

Hunger / Cravings

Some

None   Intense

Hydration

Today's Weight

Notes / Observations

....
....
....
....
....
....
....
....
....
....

Today I Feel...

Sleep Quality

Sleep Time

_____

Wake Time

_____

Date: _____   Fasting Day?   Y   N

		MACROS	
BREAKFAST		Protein	
		Carbs	
		Fat	
		Calories	
LUNCH		MACROS	
		Protein	
		Carbs	
		Fat	
		Calories	
DINNER		MACROS	
		Protein	
		Carbs	
		Fat	
		Calories	
SNACKS		MACROS	
		Protein	
		Carbs	
		Fat	
		Calories	

Hunger / Cravings

Some

None   Intense

Hydration

Today's Weight

Notes / Observations

....

....

....

....

....

....

....

....

....

....

Today I Feel...

Sleep Quality

Sleep Time

_____

Wake Time

_____

Date: _____   Fasting Day?   Y   N

		MACROS	
BREAKFAST		Protein	
		Carbs	
		Fat	
		Calories	
LUNCH		MACROS	
		Protein	
		Carbs	
		Fat	
		Calories	
DINNER		MACROS	
		Protein	
		Carbs	
		Fat	
		Calories	
SNACKS		MACROS	
		Protein	
		Carbs	
		Fat	
		Calories	

Hunger / Cravings

Some

None   Intense

Hydration

Today's Weight

Notes / Observations

....

....

....

....

....

....

....

....

....

Today I Feel...

Sleep Quality

Sleep Time
_____

Wake Time
_____

Date: _____   Fasting Day?   Y   N

		MACROS	
BREAKFAST		Protein	
		Carbs	
		Fat	
		Calories	
LUNCH		MACROS	
		Protein	
		Carbs	
		Fat	
		Calories	
DINNER		MACROS	
		Protein	
		Carbs	
		Fat	
		Calories	
SNACKS		MACROS	
		Protein	
		Carbs	
		Fat	
		Calories	

Hunger / Cravings

Some

None   Intense

Hydration

Today's Weight

Notes / Observations

....

....

....

....

....

....

....

....

....

Today I Feel...

Sleep Quality

Sleep Time
_____

Wake Time
_____

Date: _____   Fasting Day?   Y   N

	MACROS	
BREAKFAST	Protein	
	Carbs	
	Fat	
	Calories	
	MACROS	
LUNCH	Protein	
	Carbs	
	Fat	
	Calories	
	MACROS	
DINNER	Protein	
	Carbs	
	Fat	
	Calories	
	MACROS	
SNACKS	Protein	
	Carbs	
	Fat	
	Calories	

Hunger / Cravings

Some
None   Intense

Hydration

Today's Weight

Notes / Observations

....
....
....
....
....
....
....
....

Today I Feel...

Sleep Quality

Sleep Time
_____

Wake Time
_____

Date: _____   Fasting Day?   Y   N

		MACROS	
BREAKFAST		Protein	
		Carbs	
		Fat	
		Calories	
LUNCH		MACROS	
		Protein	
		Carbs	
		Fat	
		Calories	
DINNER		MACROS	
		Protein	
		Carbs	
		Fat	
		Calories	
SNACKS		MACROS	
		Protein	
		Carbs	
		Fat	
		Calories	

Hunger / Cravings

Some

None   Intense

Hydration

Today's Weight

Notes / Observations

....

....

....

....

....

....

....

....

....

....

Today I Feel...

Sleep Quality

Sleep Time

_____

Wake Time

_____

Date: _____ Fasting Day?   Y   N

		MACROS	
BREAKFAST		Protein	
		Carbs	
		Fat	
		Calories	
LUNCH		MACROS	
		Protein	
		Carbs	
		Fat	
		Calories	
DINNER		MACROS	
		Protein	
		Carbs	
		Fat	
		Calories	
SNACKS		MACROS	
		Protein	
		Carbs	
		Fat	
		Calories	

Hunger / Cravings

Some

None

Intense

Hydration

Today's Weight

Notes / Observations

....
....
....
....
....
....
....
....
....

Today I Feel...

Sleep Quality

Sleep Time

_____

Wake Time

_____

Date: _____ Fasting Day?   Y   N

		MACROS	
BREAKFAST		Protein	
		Carbs	
		Fat	
		Calories	
LUNCH		MACROS	
		Protein	
		Carbs	
		Fat	
		Calories	
DINNER		MACROS	
		Protein	
		Carbs	
		Fat	
		Calories	
SNACKS		MACROS	
		Protein	
		Carbs	
		Fat	
		Calories	

Hunger / Cravings

Some
None   Intense

Hydration

Today's Weight

Notes / Observations

....
....
....
....
....
....
....
....
....
....

Today I Feel...

Sleep Quality

Sleep Time

_____

Wake Time

_____

Date: _____ Fasting Day?   Y   N

		MACROS	
BREAKFAST		Protein	
		Carbs	
		Fat	
		Calories	
LUNCH		MACROS	
		Protein	
		Carbs	
		Fat	
		Calories	
DINNER		MACROS	
		Protein	
		Carbs	
		Fat	
		Calories	
SNACKS		MACROS	
		Protein	
		Carbs	
		Fat	
		Calories	

Hunger / Cravings

Some

None   Intense

Hydration

Today's Weight

Notes / Observations

....
....
....
....
....
....
....
....
....
....

Today I Feel...

Sleep Quality

Sleep Time
_____

Wake Time
_____

Date: _____   Fasting Day?   Y   N

		MACROS	
BREAKFAST		Protein	
		Carbs	
		Fat	
		Calories	
LUNCH		MACROS	
		Protein	
		Carbs	
		Fat	
		Calories	
DINNER		MACROS	
		Protein	
		Carbs	
		Fat	
		Calories	
SNACKS		MACROS	
		Protein	
		Carbs	
		Fat	
		Calories	

Hunger / Cravings

Hydration

Today's Weight

Notes / Observations

....
....
....
....
....
....
....
....
....
....

Today I Feel...

Sleep Quality

Sleep Time _____

Wake Time _____

Date: _____   Fasting Day?   Y   N

		MACROS	
BREAKFAST		Protein	
		Carbs	
		Fat	
		Calories	
LUNCH		MACROS	
		Protein	
		Carbs	
		Fat	
		Calories	
DINNER		MACROS	
		Protein	
		Carbs	
		Fat	
		Calories	
SNACKS		MACROS	
		Protein	
		Carbs	
		Fat	
		Calories	

Hunger / Cravings

Some

None   Intense

Hydration

Today's Weight

Notes / Observations

....

....

....

....

....

....

....

....

Today I Feel...

Sleep Quality

Sleep Time

_____

Wake Time

_____

Date: _____   Fasting Day?   Y   N

		MACROS	
BREAKFAST		Protein	
		Carbs	
		Fat	
		Calories	
LUNCH		MACROS	
		Protein	
		Carbs	
		Fat	
		Calories	
DINNER		MACROS	
		Protein	
		Carbs	
		Fat	
		Calories	
SNACKS		MACROS	
		Protein	
		Carbs	
		Fat	
		Calories	

Hunger / Cravings

Some

None   Intense

Hydration

Today's Weight

Notes / Observations

....
....
....
....
....
....
....
....
....

Today I Feel...

Sleep Quality

Sleep Time

_____

Wake Time

_____

Date: _____   Fasting Day?   Y   N

		MACROS	
BREAKFAST		Protein	
		Carbs	
		Fat	
		Calories	
LUNCH		MACROS	
		Protein	
		Carbs	
		Fat	
		Calories	
DINNER		MACROS	
		Protein	
		Carbs	
		Fat	
		Calories	
SNACKS		MACROS	
		Protein	
		Carbs	
		Fat	
		Calories	

Hunger / Cravings

Some

None   Intense

Hydration

Today's Weight

Notes / Observations

....
....
....
....
....
....
....
....
....

Today I Feel...

Sleep Quality

Sleep Time
_____

Wake Time
_____

Date: _____   Fasting Day?   Y   N

		MACROS	
BREAKFAST		Protein	
		Carbs	
		Fat	
		Calories	
LUNCH		MACROS	
		Protein	
		Carbs	
		Fat	
		Calories	
DINNER		MACROS	
		Protein	
		Carbs	
		Fat	
		Calories	
SNACKS		MACROS	
		Protein	
		Carbs	
		Fat	
		Calories	

Hunger / Cravings

Some
None   Intense

Hydration

Today's Weight

Notes / Observations

....
....
....
....
....
....
....
....
....

Today I Feel...

Sleep Quality

Sleep Time
_____

Wake Time
_____

Date: _____   Fasting Day?   Y   N

		MACROS	
BREAKFAST		Protein	
		Carbs	
		Fat	
		Calories	
LUNCH		MACROS	
		Protein	
		Carbs	
		Fat	
		Calories	
DINNER		MACROS	
		Protein	
		Carbs	
		Fat	
		Calories	
SNACKS		MACROS	
		Protein	
		Carbs	
		Fat	
		Calories	

Hunger / Cravings

Some
None   Intense

Hydration

Today's Weight

Notes / Observations

....
....
....
....
....
....
....
....
....
....

Today I Feel...

Sleep Quality

Sleep Time
_____

Wake Time
_____

Date: _____ Fasting Day?   Y   N

		MACROS	
BREAKFAST		Protein	
		Carbs	
		Fat	
		Calories	
LUNCH		MACROS	
		Protein	
		Carbs	
		Fat	
		Calories	
DINNER		MACROS	
		Protein	
		Carbs	
		Fat	
		Calories	
SNACKS		MACROS	
		Protein	
		Carbs	
		Fat	
		Calories	

Hunger / Cravings

Some

None   Intense

Hydration

Today's Weight

Notes / Observations

....

....

....

....

....

....

....

....

....

....

Today I Feel...

Sleep Quality

Sleep Time

_____

Wake Time

_____

Date: _____   Fasting Day?   Y   N

		MACROS	
BREAKFAST		Protein	
		Carbs	
		Fat	
		Calories	
LUNCH		MACROS	
		Protein	
		Carbs	
		Fat	
		Calories	
DINNER		MACROS	
		Protein	
		Carbs	
		Fat	
		Calories	
SNACKS		MACROS	
		Protein	
		Carbs	
		Fat	
		Calories	

Hunger / Cravings

Some

None   Intense

Hydration

Today's Weight

Notes / Observations

....
....
....
....
....
....
....
....
....

Today I Feel...

Sleep Quality

Sleep Time
_____

Wake Time
_____

Date: _____   Fasting Day?   Y   N

		MACROS	
BREAKFAST		Protein	
		Carbs	
		Fat	
		Calories	
LUNCH		MACROS	
		Protein	
		Carbs	
		Fat	
		Calories	
DINNER		MACROS	
		Protein	
		Carbs	
		Fat	
		Calories	
SNACKS		MACROS	
		Protein	
		Carbs	
		Fat	
		Calories	

Hunger / Cravings

Some
None   Intense

Hydration

Today's Weight

Notes / Observations

....
....
....
....
....
....
....
....
....
....

Today I Feel...

Sleep Quality

Sleep Time

_____

Wake Time

_____

Date: _____ Fasting Day?   Y   N

BREAKFAST		Macros	
		Protein	
		Carbs	
		Fat	
		Calories	

LUNCH		Macros	
		Protein	
		Carbs	
		Fat	
		Calories	

DINNER		Macros	
		Protein	
		Carbs	
		Fat	
		Calories	

SNACKS		Macros	
		Protein	
		Carbs	
		Fat	
		Calories	

Hunger / Cravings

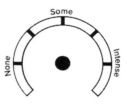

Hydration

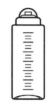

Today's Weight

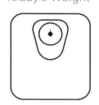

Notes / Observations

....
....
....
....
....
....
....
....
....
....

Today I Feel...

Sleep Quality

Sleep Time

_____

Wake Time

_____

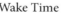

Date: _____   Fasting Day?   Y   N

BREAKFAST		MACROS	
		Protein	
		Carbs	
		Fat	
		Calories	

LUNCH		MACROS	
		Protein	
		Carbs	
		Fat	
		Calories	

DINNER		MACROS	
		Protein	
		Carbs	
		Fat	
		Calories	

SNACKS		MACROS	
		Protein	
		Carbs	
		Fat	
		Calories	

Hunger / Cravings

Hydration

Today's Weight

Notes / Observations

....
....
....
....
....
....
....
....
....

Today I Feel...

Sleep Quality

Sleep Time

_____

Wake Time

_____

Date: _____   Fasting Day?   Y   N

		MACROS	
BREAKFAST		Protein	
		Carbs	
		Fat	
		Calories	
LUNCH		MACROS	
		Protein	
		Carbs	
		Fat	
		Calories	
DINNER		MACROS	
		Protein	
		Carbs	
		Fat	
		Calories	
SNACKS		MACROS	
		Protein	
		Carbs	
		Fat	
		Calories	

Hunger / Cravings

Some

None   Intense

Hydration

Today's Weight

Notes / Observations

....
....
....
....
....
....
....
....
....

Today I Feel...

Sleep Quality

Sleep Time
_____

Wake Time
_____

Date: _____ Fasting Day?   Y   N

		MACROS	
BREAKFAST		Protein	
		Carbs	
		Fat	
		Calories	
LUNCH		MACROS	
		Protein	
		Carbs	
		Fat	
		Calories	
DINNER		MACROS	
		Protein	
		Carbs	
		Fat	
		Calories	
SNACKS		MACROS	
		Protein	
		Carbs	
		Fat	
		Calories	

Hunger / Cravings

Some

None   Intense

Hydration

Today's Weight

Notes / Observations

....

....

....

....

....

....

....

....

....

....

Today I Feel...

Sleep Quality

Sleep Time

_____

Wake Time

_____

Date: _____   Fasting Day?   Y   N

BREAKFAST		Macros	
		Protein	
		Carbs	
		Fat	
		Calories	
LUNCH		Macros	
		Protein	
		Carbs	
		Fat	
		Calories	
DINNER		Macros	
		Protein	
		Carbs	
		Fat	
		Calories	
SNACKS		Macros	
		Protein	
		Carbs	
		Fat	
		Calories	

Hunger / Cravings

Some
None   Intense

Hydration

Today's Weight

Notes / Observations

....
....
....
....
....
....
....
....
....

Today I Feel...

Sleep Quality

Sleep Time

_____

Wake Time

_____

Date: _____   Fasting Day?   Y   N

		MACROS	
BREAKFAST		Protein	
		Carbs	
		Fat	
		Calories	
LUNCH		MACROS	
		Protein	
		Carbs	
		Fat	
		Calories	
DINNER		MACROS	
		Protein	
		Carbs	
		Fat	
		Calories	
SNACKS		MACROS	
		Protein	
		Carbs	
		Fat	
		Calories	

Hunger / Cravings

Some
None
Intense

Hydration

Today's Weight

Notes / Observations

....
....
....
....
....
....
....
....
....
....

Today I Feel...

Sleep Quality

Sleep Time
_____

Wake Time
_____

Date: _____   Fasting Day?   Y   N

BREAKFAST		Macros	
		Protein	
		Carbs	
		Fat	
		Calories	

LUNCH		Macros	
		Protein	
		Carbs	
		Fat	
		Calories	

DINNER		Macros	
		Protein	
		Carbs	
		Fat	
		Calories	

SNACKS		Macros	
		Protein	
		Carbs	
		Fat	
		Calories	

Hunger / Cravings

Some
None   Intense

Hydration

Today's Weight

Notes / Observations

....
....
....
....
....
....
....
....
....

Today I Feel...

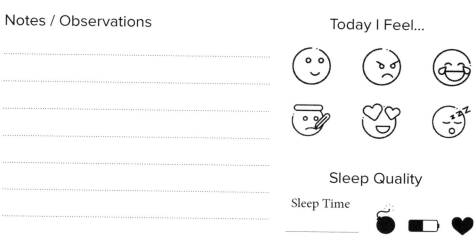

Sleep Quality

Sleep Time
_____

Wake Time
_____

Date: _____ Fasting Day?   Y   N

BREAKFAST		MACROS	
		Protein	
		Carbs	
		Fat	
		Calories	
LUNCH		MACROS	
		Protein	
		Carbs	
		Fat	
		Calories	
DINNER		MACROS	
		Protein	
		Carbs	
		Fat	
		Calories	
SNACKS		MACROS	
		Protein	
		Carbs	
		Fat	
		Calories	

Hunger / Cravings

Hydration

Today's Weight

Notes / Observations

....

....

....

....

....

....

....

....

....

Today I Feel...

Sleep Quality

Sleep Time

Wake Time

Date: _____ Fasting Day?   Y   N

		MACROS	
BREAKFAST		Protein	
		Carbs	
		Fat	
		Calories	
LUNCH		MACROS	
		Protein	
		Carbs	
		Fat	
		Calories	
DINNER		MACROS	
		Protein	
		Carbs	
		Fat	
		Calories	
SNACKS		MACROS	
		Protein	
		Carbs	
		Fat	
		Calories	

Hunger / Cravings

Some

None   Intense

Hydration

Today's Weight

Notes / Observations

....
....
....
....
....
....
....
....
....
....

Today I Feel...

Sleep Quality

Sleep Time

_____

Wake Time

_____

Date: _____   Fasting Day?   Y   N

		MACROS	
BREAKFAST		Protein	
		Carbs	
		Fat	
		Calories	
LUNCH		MACROS	
		Protein	
		Carbs	
		Fat	
		Calories	
DINNER		MACROS	
		Protein	
		Carbs	
		Fat	
		Calories	
SNACKS		MACROS	
		Protein	
		Carbs	
		Fat	
		Calories	

Hunger / Cravings

None   Some   Intense

Hydration

Today's Weight

Notes / Observations

....

....

....

....

....

....

....

....

....

Today I Feel...

Sleep Quality

Sleep Time
_____

Wake Time
_____

Date: _____   Fasting Day?   Y   N

	MACROS	
BREAKFAST	Protein	
	Carbs	
	Fat	
	Calories	
	MACROS	
LUNCH	Protein	
	Carbs	
	Fat	
	Calories	
	MACROS	
DINNER	Protein	
	Carbs	
	Fat	
	Calories	
	MACROS	
SNACKS	Protein	
	Carbs	
	Fat	
	Calories	

Hunger / Cravings

Some

None   Intense

Hydration

Today's Weight

Notes / Observations

....
....
....
....
....
....
....
....
....
....
....
....

Today I Feel...

Sleep Quality

Sleep Time

_____

Wake Time

_____

Date: _____   Fasting Day?   Y   N

		MACROS	
BREAKFAST		Protein	
		Carbs	
		Fat	
		Calories	
LUNCH		MACROS	
		Protein	
		Carbs	
		Fat	
		Calories	
DINNER		MACROS	
		Protein	
		Carbs	
		Fat	
		Calories	
SNACKS		MACROS	
		Protein	
		Carbs	
		Fat	
		Calories	

Hunger / Cravings

Some
None   Intense

Hydration

Today's Weight

Notes / Observations

Today I Feel...

Sleep Quality

Sleep Time
_____

Wake Time
_____

Date: _____   Fasting Day?   Y   N

BREAKFAST		MACROS	
		Protein	
		Carbs	
		Fat	
		Calories	

LUNCH		MACROS	
		Protein	
		Carbs	
		Fat	
		Calories	

DINNER		MACROS	
		Protein	
		Carbs	
		Fat	
		Calories	

SNACKS		MACROS	
		Protein	
		Carbs	
		Fat	
		Calories	

Hunger / Cravings

Some
None   Intense

Hydration

Today's Weight

Notes / Observations

....
....
....
....
....
....
....
....
....

Today I Feel...

Sleep Quality

Sleep Time
_____

Wake Time
_____

Date: _____ Fasting Day? Y N

		MACROS	
BREAKFAST		Protein	
		Carbs	
		Fat	
		Calories	
LUNCH		MACROS	
		Protein	
		Carbs	
		Fat	
		Calories	
DINNER		MACROS	
		Protein	
		Carbs	
		Fat	
		Calories	
SNACKS		MACROS	
		Protein	
		Carbs	
		Fat	
		Calories	

Hunger / Cravings

Some
None   Intense

Hydration

Today's Weight

Notes / Observations

....
....
....
....
....
....
....
....
....

Today I Feel...

Sleep Quality

Sleep Time
_____

Wake Time
_____

Date: _____   Fasting Day?   Y   N

		MACROS	
BREAKFAST		Protein	
		Carbs	
		Fat	
		Calories	
LUNCH		MACROS	
		Protein	
		Carbs	
		Fat	
		Calories	
DINNER		MACROS	
		Protein	
		Carbs	
		Fat	
		Calories	
SNACKS		MACROS	
		Protein	
		Carbs	
		Fat	
		Calories	

Hunger / Cravings

Some

None   Intense

Hydration

Today's Weight

Notes / Observations

....
....
....
....
....
....
....
....
....

Today I Feel...

Sleep Quality

Sleep Time

_____

Wake Time

_____

Date: _____   Fasting Day?   Y   N

	MACROS	
BREAKFAST	Protein	
	Carbs	
	Fat	
	Calories	
	MACROS	
LUNCH	Protein	
	Carbs	
	Fat	
	Calories	
	MACROS	
DINNER	Protein	
	Carbs	
	Fat	
	Calories	
	MACROS	
SNACKS	Protein	
	Carbs	
	Fat	
	Calories	

Hunger / Cravings

Some

None   Intense

Hydration

Today's Weight

Notes / Observations

....

....

....

....

....

....

....

....

....

Today I Feel...

Sleep Quality

Sleep Time

_____

Wake Time

_____

Date: _____   Fasting Day?   Y   N

BREAKFAST		Macros	
		Protein	
		Carbs	
		Fat	
		Calories	
LUNCH		Macros	
		Protein	
		Carbs	
		Fat	
		Calories	
DINNER		Macros	
		Protein	
		Carbs	
		Fat	
		Calories	
SNACKS		Macros	
		Protein	
		Carbs	
		Fat	
		Calories	

Hunger / Cravings

Some
None   Intense

Hydration

Today's Weight

Notes / Observations

....
....
....
....
....
....
....
....
....

Today I Feel...

Sleep Quality

Sleep Time

_____

Wake Time

_____

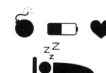

Date: _____   Fasting Day?   Y   N

BREAKFAST		Macros	
		Protein	
		Carbs	
		Fat	
		Calories	

LUNCH		Macros	
		Protein	
		Carbs	
		Fat	
		Calories	

DINNER		Macros	
		Protein	
		Carbs	
		Fat	
		Calories	

SNACKS		Macros	
		Protein	
		Carbs	
		Fat	
		Calories	

Hunger / Cravings

Some
None   Intense

Hydration

Today's Weight

Notes / Observations

....
....
....
....
....
....
....
....

Today I Feel...

Sleep Quality

Sleep Time
_____

Wake Time
_____

Date: _____   Fasting Day?   Y   N

BREAKFAST		Macros	
		Protein	
		Carbs	
		Fat	
		Calories	

LUNCH		Macros	
		Protein	
		Carbs	
		Fat	
		Calories	

DINNER		Macros	
		Protein	
		Carbs	
		Fat	
		Calories	

SNACKS		Macros	
		Protein	
		Carbs	
		Fat	
		Calories	

Hunger / Cravings

Some
None
Intense

Hydration

Today's Weight

Notes / Observations

....
....
....
....
....
....
....
....
....
....

Today I Feel...

Sleep Quality

Sleep Time

_____

Wake Time

_____

Date: _____   Fasting Day?   Y   N

		MACROS	
BREAKFAST		Protein	
		Carbs	
		Fat	
		Calories	
LUNCH		MACROS	
		Protein	
		Carbs	
		Fat	
		Calories	
DINNER		MACROS	
		Protein	
		Carbs	
		Fat	
		Calories	
SNACKS		MACROS	
		Protein	
		Carbs	
		Fat	
		Calories	

Hunger / Cravings

Some
None   Intense

Hydration

Today's Weight

Notes / Observations

....
....
....
....
....
....
....
....
....
....

Today I Feel...

Sleep Quality

Sleep Time

_____

Wake Time

_____

Date: _____   Fasting Day?   Y   N

		MACROS	
BREAKFAST		Protein	
		Carbs	
		Fat	
		Calories	
LUNCH		MACROS	
		Protein	
		Carbs	
		Fat	
		Calories	
DINNER		MACROS	
		Protein	
		Carbs	
		Fat	
		Calories	
SNACKS		MACROS	
		Protein	
		Carbs	
		Fat	
		Calories	

Hunger / Cravings

Some
None   Intense

Hydration

Today's Weight

Notes / Observations

....
....
....
....
....
....
....
....
....
....

Today I Feel...

Sleep Quality

Sleep Time

_____

Wake Time

_____

Date: _____   Fasting Day?   Y   N

		MACROS	
BREAKFAST		Protein	
		Carbs	
		Fat	
		Calories	
LUNCH		MACROS	
		Protein	
		Carbs	
		Fat	
		Calories	
DINNER		MACROS	
		Protein	
		Carbs	
		Fat	
		Calories	
SNACKS		MACROS	
		Protein	
		Carbs	
		Fat	
		Calories	

Hunger / Cravings

Some
None — Intense

Hydration

Today's Weight

Notes / Observations

....
....
....
....
....
....
....
....
....

Today I Feel...

Sleep Quality

Sleep Time
_____

Wake Time
_____

Date: _____   Fasting Day?   Y   N

BREAKFAST		Macros	
		Protein	
		Carbs	
		Fat	
		Calories	

LUNCH		Macros	
		Protein	
		Carbs	
		Fat	
		Calories	

DINNER		Macros	
		Protein	
		Carbs	
		Fat	
		Calories	

SNACKS		Macros	
		Protein	
		Carbs	
		Fat	
		Calories	

Hunger / Cravings

Some

None   Intense

Hydration

Today's Weight

Notes / Observations

....
....
....
....
....
....
....
....
....
....

Today I Feel...

Sleep Quality

Sleep Time

_____

Wake Time

Date: _____   Fasting Day?   Y   N

	MACROS	
BREAKFAST	Protein	
	Carbs	
	Fat	
	Calories	

	MACROS	
LUNCH	Protein	
	Carbs	
	Fat	
	Calories	

	MACROS	
DINNER	Protein	
	Carbs	
	Fat	
	Calories	

	MACROS	
SNACKS	Protein	
	Carbs	
	Fat	
	Calories	

Hunger / Cravings

Some

None   Intense

Hydration

Today's Weight

Notes / Observations

....

....

....

....

....

....

....

....

....

....

Today I Feel...

Sleep Quality

Sleep Time

_____

Wake Time

_____

Date: _____   Fasting Day?   Y   N

	MACROS	
BREAKFAST	Protein	
	Carbs	
	Fat	
	Calories	
	MACROS	
LUNCH	Protein	
	Carbs	
	Fat	
	Calories	
	MACROS	
DINNER	Protein	
	Carbs	
	Fat	
	Calories	
	MACROS	
SNACKS	Protein	
	Carbs	
	Fat	
	Calories	

Hunger / Cravings

Some

None   Intense

Hydration

Today's Weight

Notes / Observations

....

....

....

....

....

....

....

....

....

....

....

....

Today I Feel...

Sleep Quality

Sleep Time

_____

Wake Time

_____

Date: _____ Fasting Day?   Y   N

	MACROS	
BREAKFAST	Protein	
	Carbs	
	Fat	
	Calories	

	MACROS	
LUNCH	Protein	
	Carbs	
	Fat	
	Calories	

	MACROS	
DINNER	Protein	
	Carbs	
	Fat	
	Calories	

	MACROS	
SNACKS	Protein	
	Carbs	
	Fat	
	Calories	

Hunger / Cravings

Some
None   Intense

Hydration

Today's Weight

Notes / Observations

....

....

....

....

....

....

....

....

....

Today I Feel...

Sleep Quality

Sleep Time

_____

Wake Time

_____

Date: _____   Fasting Day?   Y   N

BREAKFAST		MACROS	
		Protein	
		Carbs	
		Fat	
		Calories	

LUNCH		MACROS	
		Protein	
		Carbs	
		Fat	
		Calories	

DINNER		MACROS	
		Protein	
		Carbs	
		Fat	
		Calories	

SNACKS		MACROS	
		Protein	
		Carbs	
		Fat	
		Calories	

Hunger / Cravings

Some
None   Intense

Hydration

Today's Weight

Notes / Observations

....
....
....
....
....
....
....
....
....
....

Today I Feel...

Sleep Quality

Sleep Time

_____

Wake Time

_____

Date: _____ Fasting Day?   Y   N

		MACROS	
BREAKFAST		Protein	
		Carbs	
		Fat	
		Calories	
LUNCH		MACROS	
		Protein	
		Carbs	
		Fat	
		Calories	
DINNER		MACROS	
		Protein	
		Carbs	
		Fat	
		Calories	
SNACKS		MACROS	
		Protein	
		Carbs	
		Fat	
		Calories	

Hunger / Cravings

Some

None   Intense

Hydration

Today's Weight

Notes / Observations

....

....

....

....

....

....

....

....

....

....

Today I Feel...

Sleep Quality

Sleep Time

_____

Wake Time

_____

Date: _____   Fasting Day?   Y   N

BREAKFAST		MACROS	
		Protein	
		Carbs	
		Fat	
		Calories	

LUNCH		MACROS	
		Protein	
		Carbs	
		Fat	
		Calories	

DINNER		MACROS	
		Protein	
		Carbs	
		Fat	
		Calories	

SNACKS		MACROS	
		Protein	
		Carbs	
		Fat	
		Calories	

Hunger / Cravings

Some
None
Intense

Hydration

Today's Weight

Notes / Observations

....
....
....
....
....
....
....
....
....

Today I Feel...

Sleep Quality

Sleep Time

_____

Wake Time

_____

Date: _____   Fasting Day?   Y   N

		MACROS	
BREAKFAST		Protein	
		Carbs	
		Fat	
		Calories	
LUNCH		MACROS	
		Protein	
		Carbs	
		Fat	
		Calories	
DINNER		MACROS	
		Protein	
		Carbs	
		Fat	
		Calories	
SNACKS		MACROS	
		Protein	
		Carbs	
		Fat	
		Calories	

Hunger / Cravings

Some
None   Intense

Hydration

Today's Weight

Notes / Observations

....
....
....
....
....
....
....
....
....

Today I Feel...

Sleep Quality

Sleep Time
_____

Wake Time
_____

Date: _____   Fasting Day?   Y   N

	MACROS	
BREAKFAST	Protein	
	Carbs	
	Fat	
	Calories	

	MACROS	
LUNCH	Protein	
	Carbs	
	Fat	
	Calories	

	MACROS	
DINNER	Protein	
	Carbs	
	Fat	
	Calories	

	MACROS	
SNACKS	Protein	
	Carbs	
	Fat	
	Calories	

Hunger / Cravings

Some
None   Intense

Hydration

Today's Weight

Notes / Observations

....
....
....
....
....
....
....
....
....

Today I Feel...

Sleep Quality

Sleep Time
_____

Wake Time
_____

Date: _____   Fasting Day?   Y   N

		MACROS	
BREAKFAST		Protein	
		Carbs	
		Fat	
		Calories	
LUNCH		MACROS	
		Protein	
		Carbs	
		Fat	
		Calories	
DINNER		MACROS	
		Protein	
		Carbs	
		Fat	
		Calories	
SNACKS		MACROS	
		Protein	
		Carbs	
		Fat	
		Calories	

Hunger / Cravings

Some
None   Intense

Hydration

Today's Weight

Notes / Observations

....
....
....
....
....
....
....
....
....
....

Today I Feel...

Sleep Quality

Sleep Time
_____

Wake Time
_____

Date: _____   Fasting Day?   Y   N

	MACROS	
BREAKFAST	Protein	
	Carbs	
	Fat	
	Calories	

	MACROS	
LUNCH	Protein	
	Carbs	
	Fat	
	Calories	

	MACROS	
DINNER	Protein	
	Carbs	
	Fat	
	Calories	

	MACROS	
SNACKS	Protein	
	Carbs	
	Fat	
	Calories	

Hunger / Cravings

Hydration

Today's Weight

Notes / Observations

....
....
....
....
....
....
....
....
....

Today I Feel...

Sleep Quality

Sleep Time

_____

Wake Time

_____

Date: _____ Fasting Day? Y   N

		MACROS	
BREAKFAST		Protein	
		Carbs	
		Fat	
		Calories	
LUNCH		MACROS	
		Protein	
		Carbs	
		Fat	
		Calories	
DINNER		MACROS	
		Protein	
		Carbs	
		Fat	
		Calories	
SNACKS		MACROS	
		Protein	
		Carbs	
		Fat	
		Calories	

Hunger / Cravings

Some

None   Intense

Hydration

Today's Weight

Notes / Observations

....

....

....

....

....

....

....

....

....

Today I Feel...

Sleep Quality

Sleep Time

_____

Wake Time

_____

Date: _____   Fasting Day?   Y   N

	MACROS	
BREAKFAST	Protein	
	Carbs	
	Fat	
	Calories	

	MACROS	
LUNCH	Protein	
	Carbs	
	Fat	
	Calories	

	MACROS	
DINNER	Protein	
	Carbs	
	Fat	
	Calories	

	MACROS	
SNACKS	Protein	
	Carbs	
	Fat	
	Calories	

Hunger / Cravings

Some

None   Intense

Hydration

Today's Weight

Notes / Observations

....
....
....
....
....
....
....
....
....
....

Today I Feel...

Sleep Quality

Sleep Time

_____

Wake Time

_____

Date: _____ Fasting Day?   Y   N

	MACROS	
BREAKFAST	Protein	
	Carbs	
	Fat	
	Calories	

	MACROS	
LUNCH	Protein	
	Carbs	
	Fat	
	Calories	

	MACROS	
DINNER	Protein	
	Carbs	
	Fat	
	Calories	

	MACROS	
SNACKS	Protein	
	Carbs	
	Fat	
	Calories	

Hunger / Cravings

Some
None   Intense

Hydration

Today's Weight

Notes / Observations

....
....
....
....
....
....
....
....
....

Today I Feel...

Sleep Quality

Sleep Time
_____

Wake Time

Date: _____   Fasting Day?   Y   N

BREAKFAST		Macros	
		Protein	
		Carbs	
		Fat	
		Calories	

LUNCH		Macros	
		Protein	
		Carbs	
		Fat	
		Calories	

DINNER		Macros	
		Protein	
		Carbs	
		Fat	
		Calories	

SNACKS		Macros	
		Protein	
		Carbs	
		Fat	
		Calories	

Hunger / Cravings

Some
None   Intense

Hydration

Today's Weight

Notes / Observations

....
....
....
....
....
....
....
....
....

Today I Feel...

Sleep Quality

Sleep Time
_____

Wake Time
_____

Date: _____   Fasting Day?   Y   N

BREAKFAST		MACROS	
		Protein	
		Carbs	
		Fat	
		Calories	

LUNCH		MACROS	
		Protein	
		Carbs	
		Fat	
		Calories	

DINNER		MACROS	
		Protein	
		Carbs	
		Fat	
		Calories	

SNACKS		MACROS	
		Protein	
		Carbs	
		Fat	
		Calories	

Hunger / Cravings

Hydration

Today's Weight

Notes / Observations

....
....
....
....
....
....
....
....
....

Today I Feel...

Sleep Quality

Sleep Time

_____

Wake Time

_____

Date: _____   Fasting Day?   Y   N

		MACROS	
BREAKFAST		Protein	
		Carbs	
		Fat	
		Calories	
LUNCH		MACROS	
		Protein	
		Carbs	
		Fat	
		Calories	
DINNER		MACROS	
		Protein	
		Carbs	
		Fat	
		Calories	
SNACKS		MACROS	
		Protein	
		Carbs	
		Fat	
		Calories	

Hunger / Cravings

Some

None   Intense

Hydration

Today's Weight

Notes / Observations

....

....

....

....

....

....

....

....

....

....

Today I Feel...

Sleep Quality

Sleep Time

_____

Wake Time

_____

z Z z

Date: _____   Fasting Day?   Y   N

		MACROS	
BREAKFAST		Protein	
		Carbs	
		Fat	
		Calories	
LUNCH		MACROS	
		Protein	
		Carbs	
		Fat	
		Calories	
DINNER		MACROS	
		Protein	
		Carbs	
		Fat	
		Calories	
SNACKS		MACROS	
		Protein	
		Carbs	
		Fat	
		Calories	

Hunger / Cravings

Some
None
Intense

Hydration

Today's Weight

Notes / Observations

....

....

....

....

....

....

....

....

....

Today I Feel...

Sleep Quality

Sleep Time

_____

Wake Time

_____

Date: _____   Fasting Day?   Y   N

	MACROS	
BREAKFAST	Protein	
	Carbs	
	Fat	
	Calories	

	MACROS	
LUNCH	Protein	
	Carbs	
	Fat	
	Calories	

	MACROS	
DINNER	Protein	
	Carbs	
	Fat	
	Calories	

	MACROS	
SNACKS	Protein	
	Carbs	
	Fat	
	Calories	

Hunger / Cravings

Some
None   Intense

Hydration

Today's Weight

Notes / Observations

....
....
....
....
....
....
....
....
....
....

Today I Feel...

Sleep Quality

Sleep Time

_____

Wake Time

_____

Date: _____ Fasting Day?   Y   N

	MACROS	
BREAKFAST	Protein	
	Carbs	
	Fat	
	Calories	
	MACROS	
LUNCH	Protein	
	Carbs	
	Fat	
	Calories	
	MACROS	
DINNER	Protein	
	Carbs	
	Fat	
	Calories	
	MACROS	
SNACKS	Protein	
	Carbs	
	Fat	
	Calories	

Hunger / Cravings

Some
None   Intense

Hydration

Today's Weight

Notes / Observations

....
....
....
....
....
....
....
....
....
....

Today I Feel...

Sleep Quality

Sleep Time
_____

Wake Time
_____

Date: _____   Fasting Day?   Y   N

	MACROS	
BREAKFAST		
	Protein	
	Carbs	
	Fat	
	Calories	

	MACROS	
LUNCH		
	Protein	
	Carbs	
	Fat	
	Calories	

	MACROS	
DINNER		
	Protein	
	Carbs	
	Fat	
	Calories	

	MACROS	
SNACKS		
	Protein	
	Carbs	
	Fat	
	Calories	

Hunger / Cravings

Some
None   Intense

Hydration

Today's Weight

Notes / Observations

....
....
....
....
....
....
....
....
....
....

Today I Feel...

Sleep Quality

Sleep Time

_____

Wake Time

_____

Date: _____ Fasting Day?   Y   N

		MACROS	
BREAKFAST		Protein	
		Carbs	
		Fat	
		Calories	
LUNCH		MACROS	
		Protein	
		Carbs	
		Fat	
		Calories	
DINNER		MACROS	
		Protein	
		Carbs	
		Fat	
		Calories	
SNACKS		MACROS	
		Protein	
		Carbs	
		Fat	
		Calories	

Hunger / Cravings

Some

None   Intense

Hydration

Today's Weight

Notes / Observations

....
....
....
....
....
....
....
....
....
....

Today I Feel...

Sleep Quality

Sleep Time

_____

Wake Time

_____

Date: _____   Fasting Day?   Y   N

	MACROS	
BREAKFAST	Protein	
	Carbs	
	Fat	
	Calories	

	MACROS	
LUNCH	Protein	
	Carbs	
	Fat	
	Calories	

	MACROS	
DINNER	Protein	
	Carbs	
	Fat	
	Calories	

	MACROS	
SNACKS	Protein	
	Carbs	
	Fat	
	Calories	

Hunger / Cravings

Some

None   Intense

Hydration

Today's Weight

Notes / Observations

....
....
....
....
....
....
....
....
....
....

Today I Feel...

Sleep Quality

Sleep Time
_____

Wake Time
_____

Date: _____   Fasting Day?   Y   N

		MACROS	
BREAKFAST		Protein	
		Carbs	
		Fat	
		Calories	
LUNCH		MACROS	
		Protein	
		Carbs	
		Fat	
		Calories	
DINNER		MACROS	
		Protein	
		Carbs	
		Fat	
		Calories	
SNACKS		MACROS	
		Protein	
		Carbs	
		Fat	
		Calories	

Hunger / Cravings

Some

None   Intense

Hydration

Today's Weight

Notes / Observations

....

....

....

....

....

....

....

....

....

Today I Feel...

Sleep Quality

Sleep Time

_____

Wake Time

_____

Date: _____ Fasting Day? Y N

BREAKFAST		MACROS	
		Protein	
		Carbs	
		Fat	
		Calories	

LUNCH		MACROS	
		Protein	
		Carbs	
		Fat	
		Calories	

DINNER		MACROS	
		Protein	
		Carbs	
		Fat	
		Calories	

SNACKS		MACROS	
		Protein	
		Carbs	
		Fat	
		Calories	

Hunger / Cravings

Some
None
Intense

Hydration

Today's Weight

Notes / Observations

....
....
....
....
....
....
....
....
....

Today I Feel...

Sleep Quality

Sleep Time
_____

Wake Time
_____

z Z
z

Date: _____ Fasting Day? Y   N

		MACROS	
BREAKFAST		Protein	
		Carbs	
		Fat	
		Calories	
LUNCH		MACROS	
		Protein	
		Carbs	
		Fat	
		Calories	
DINNER		MACROS	
		Protein	
		Carbs	
		Fat	
		Calories	
SNACKS		MACROS	
		Protein	
		Carbs	
		Fat	
		Calories	

Hunger / Cravings

Some
None   Intense

Hydration

Today's Weight

Notes / Observations

....
....
....
....
....
....
....
....
....

Today I Feel...

Sleep Quality

Sleep Time
_____

Wake Time
_____

Date: _____   Fasting Day?   Y   N

		MACROS	
BREAKFAST		Protein	
		Carbs	
		Fat	
		Calories	
LUNCH		MACROS	
		Protein	
		Carbs	
		Fat	
		Calories	
DINNER		MACROS	
		Protein	
		Carbs	
		Fat	
		Calories	
SNACKS		MACROS	
		Protein	
		Carbs	
		Fat	
		Calories	

Hunger / Cravings

None   Some   Intense

Hydration

Today's Weight

Notes / Observations

....
....
....
....
....
....
....
....
....
....

Today I Feel...

Sleep Quality

Sleep Time
_____

Wake Time
_____

Date: _____   Fasting Day?   Y   N

	MACROS	
BREAKFAST	Protein	
	Carbs	
	Fat	
	Calories	
	MACROS	
LUNCH	Protein	
	Carbs	
	Fat	
	Calories	
	MACROS	
DINNER	Protein	
	Carbs	
	Fat	
	Calories	
	MACROS	
SNACKS	Protein	
	Carbs	
	Fat	
	Calories	

Hunger / Cravings

Hydration

Today's Weight

Notes / Observations

....
....
....
....
....
....
....
....
....
....

Today I Feel...

Sleep Quality

Sleep Time
_____

Wake Time
_____

Date: _____   Fasting Day?   Y   N

BREAKFAST		Macros	
		Protein	
		Carbs	
		Fat	
		Calories	

LUNCH		Macros	
		Protein	
		Carbs	
		Fat	
		Calories	

DINNER		Macros	
		Protein	
		Carbs	
		Fat	
		Calories	

SNACKS		Macros	
		Protein	
		Carbs	
		Fat	
		Calories	

Hunger / Cravings

Some
None   Intense

Hydration

Today's Weight

Notes / Observations

....
....
....
....
....
....
....
....
....

Today I Feel...

Sleep Quality

Sleep Time
_____

Wake Time
_____

Date: _____ Fasting Day? Y N

		MACROS	
BREAKFAST		Protein	
		Carbs	
		Fat	
		Calories	
LUNCH		MACROS	
		Protein	
		Carbs	
		Fat	
		Calories	
DINNER		MACROS	
		Protein	
		Carbs	
		Fat	
		Calories	
SNACKS		MACROS	
		Protein	
		Carbs	
		Fat	
		Calories	

Hunger / Cravings

Some
None
Intense

Hydration

Today's Weight

Notes / Observations

Today I Feel...

Sleep Quality

Sleep Time
_____

Wake Time
_____

Date: _____   Fasting Day?   Y   N

	MACROS	
BREAKFAST	Protein	
	Carbs	
	Fat	
	Calories	
	MACROS	
LUNCH	Protein	
	Carbs	
	Fat	
	Calories	
	MACROS	
DINNER	Protein	
	Carbs	
	Fat	
	Calories	
	MACROS	
SNACKS	Protein	
	Carbs	
	Fat	
	Calories	

Hunger / Cravings

Some

None   Intense

Hydration

Today's Weight

Notes / Observations

....

....

....

....

....

....

....

....

....

Today I Feel...

Sleep Quality

Sleep Time

_____

Wake Time

_____

Date: _____   Fasting Day?   Y   N

		MACROS	
BREAKFAST		Protein	
		Carbs	
		Fat	
		Calories	
LUNCH		MACROS	
		Protein	
		Carbs	
		Fat	
		Calories	
DINNER		MACROS	
		Protein	
		Carbs	
		Fat	
		Calories	
SNACKS		MACROS	
		Protein	
		Carbs	
		Fat	
		Calories	

Hunger / Cravings

Some
None   Intense

Hydration

Today's Weight

Notes / Observations

....
....
....
....
....
....
....
....
....

Today I Feel...

Sleep Quality

Sleep Time

_____

Wake Time

_____

Date: _____   Fasting Day?   Y   N

	MACROS	
BREAKFAST	Protein	
	Carbs	
	Fat	
	Calories	

	MACROS	
LUNCH	Protein	
	Carbs	
	Fat	
	Calories	

	MACROS	
DINNER	Protein	
	Carbs	
	Fat	
	Calories	

	MACROS	
SNACKS	Protein	
	Carbs	
	Fat	
	Calories	

Hunger / Cravings

Some
None   Intense

Hydration

Today's Weight

Notes / Observations

....
....
....
....
....
....
....
....
....
....
....

Today I Feel...

Sleep Quality

Sleep Time

_____

Wake Time

_____

Date: _____   Fasting Day?   Y   N

		MACROS	
BREAKFAST		Protein	
		Carbs	
		Fat	
		Calories	
LUNCH		MACROS	
		Protein	
		Carbs	
		Fat	
		Calories	
DINNER		MACROS	
		Protein	
		Carbs	
		Fat	
		Calories	
SNACKS		MACROS	
		Protein	
		Carbs	
		Fat	
		Calories	

Hunger / Cravings

Some

None   Intense

Hydration

Today's Weight

Notes / Observations

....
....
....
....
....
....
....
....
....

Today I Feel...

Sleep Quality

Sleep Time

_____

Wake Time

_____

Date: _____   Fasting Day?   Y   N

		MACROS	
BREAKFAST		Protein	
		Carbs	
		Fat	
		Calories	
LUNCH		MACROS	
		Protein	
		Carbs	
		Fat	
		Calories	
DINNER		MACROS	
		Protein	
		Carbs	
		Fat	
		Calories	
SNACKS		MACROS	
		Protein	
		Carbs	
		Fat	
		Calories	

Hunger / Cravings

Some
None   Intense

Hydration

Today's Weight

Notes / Observations

....
....
....
....
....
....
....
....

Today I Feel...

Sleep Quality

Sleep Time
_____

Wake Time
_____